ISBN: 1438201451
Copyright © 2008 Bahiga EL- Haggar.
Illustrations © 2008 Bahiga EL- Haggar.

Published by: National Health Register
Distributed by: National Health Register
P. O. Box 4014, Cheyenne, WY 82003

February 2008 in Cheyenne, Wyoming USA
http://www.thenationalhealthregister.org
E-mail: nationalhealthregister@yahoo.com

Printed in: the United States of America

For information contact the National Health Register.
        Library of Congress Cataloging

Summary
The story is about an American farmer and his animal friend. He relates his discovery of a new secret food power and how he becomes a legend. The book contains a revelation to avoid overweight boost kids' grades, and offers tools to turn resistant children to healthy eating lovers. It was inspired by the findings of "Child Early Aging" the leading condition to obesity.

Dedication

To my children and grand children

Table of Contents

Acknowledgements

My deepest appreciation goes to the guidance of Dr. B. Mawardy, who supported my work throughout the research, for her endless dedication to pediatrics, and to Tamer Riad for his absolute love of children and exceptional talent that made the electronic nutrition profiling, and the tools to early detect obesity possible. To both of you, thanks for being the force behind this book. I also offer my gratitude to the Laramie County Public Library staff for their tireless efforts to seeing this work through.

Introduction

This book stimulates kids' imagination and attracts quick learning. It features the unique adventures of an American farmer and his animal friend in a captivating storytelling of events from the past. He stumbled on a secret food power that made kids smarter, benefited his community and turned him into a legend. The book captures young readers' attention not only with colorful illustrations but with interactive tool and game-like entertainment. At the same time, it successfully engages teachers and parents in an enjoyable educational journey and offers novel techniques to master healthy eating using special food model.

Disclaimer
Information in this book is intended for educational purposes only and does not replace or substitute medical advice. Always consult your provider before starting a diet.

Once upon a time there was an American farmer called Mr. Go. He got this name because he was always busy working and traveling. He lived in a small town near a neighborhood school.

Mr. Go was kind, friendly and admired by young and old. He owned a farm and a greenhouse. He had a family that loved him so much and helped him with his farm work. He also had a son, Nelson, who was a doctor.

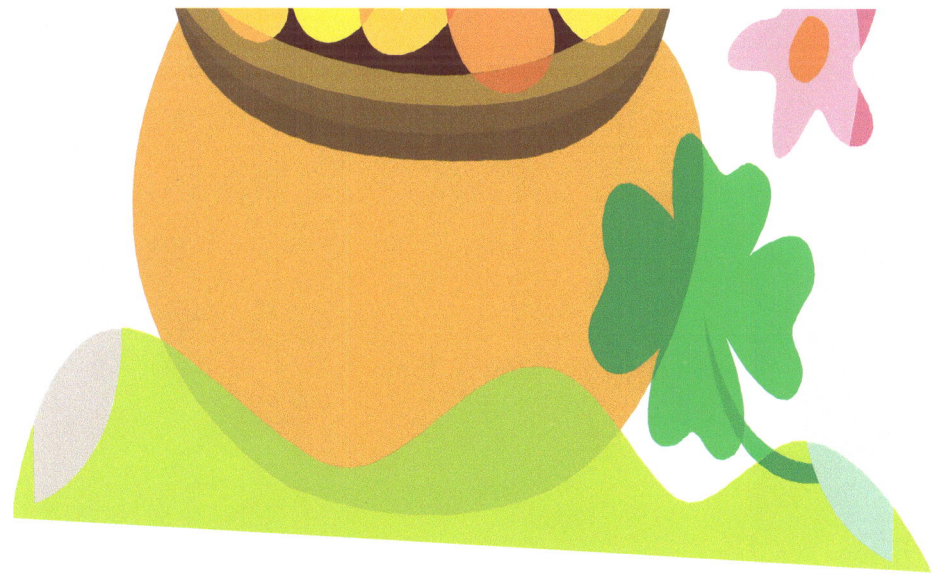

On his farm, Mr. Go planted crops for his customers. The stores in the town market paid him to grow the products that they sold.

Mr. Go loved his work because it also took him to foreign places to sell his crops. He especially enjoyed travelling. Up north, he visited Canada, and down south, he went to Mexico. He made new friends, brought home samples of exotic food and collected souvenirs.

Mr. Go had a dream that one day he would tour the wonders of the world and see the ancient ruins of Greece and the pyramids of Egypt, for example.

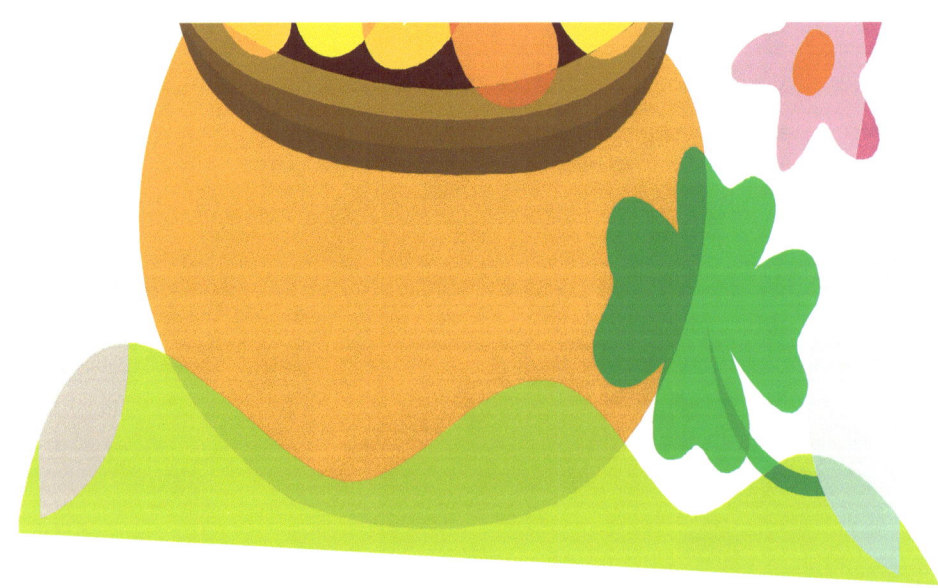

Mr. Go had an animal friend, a mule named Willie. He was extraordi-narily strong, had sharp memory and powerful hooves. Willie carried packages for Mr. Go and gave him rides whenever he needed them. Mr. Go knew that Willie was his best and long-lasting friend.

Willie would often sing a loud tune ~~HAA~~HAA~~ and happily click his hooves. The farm animals shared his joy-chickens flapped their wings, ducks quacked and chipmunks squealed. Willie was so happy that the kids thought he almost smiled.

Children loved to watch Willie sing and sometimes joined him in his musical. They called him "Clicky Hooves" Willie.

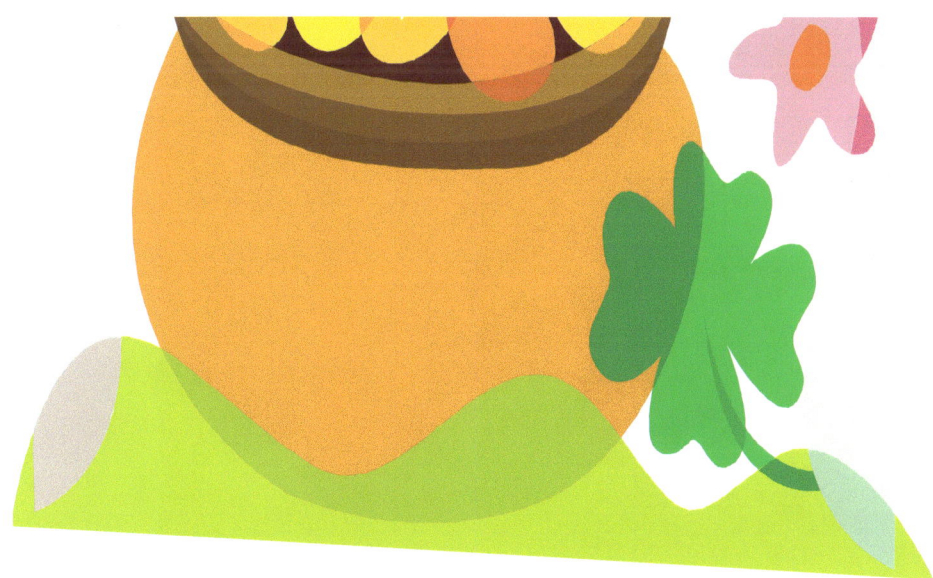

Willie had a little secret of his own, a favorite plant that grew at the corner of the farm. Mr. Go noticed that Willie got more energetic and a lot happier when he ate it.

Mr. Go told Dr. Nelson that the plant looked like beans, but he did not know it's name. He described it as thin green stems that bloomed with white flowers when in season and produced long green pods with white velvet inside liners. Each pod contained eight medium-sized beans with thick skin. The bean color turned tan when it dried.

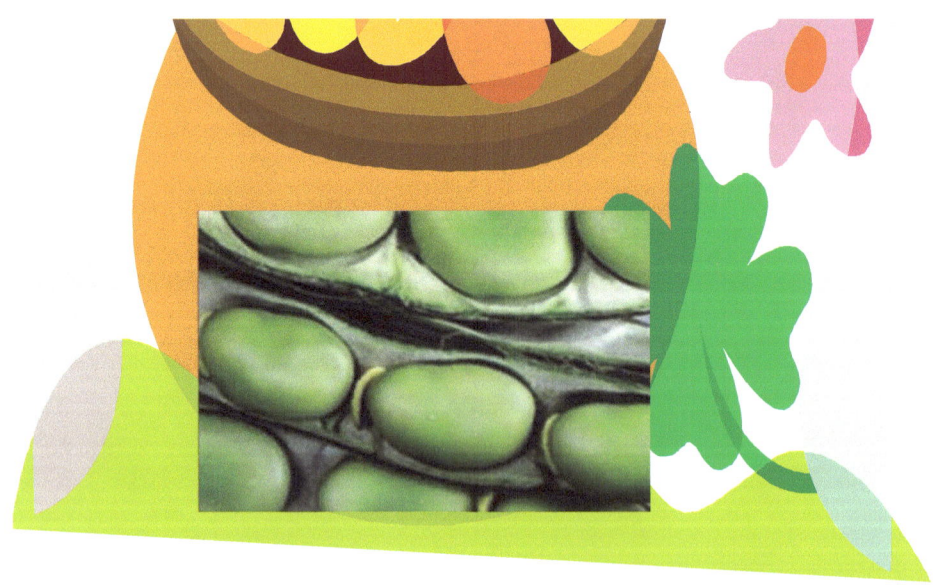

Mr. Go needed to know more about Willie's favorite food. So after work, he asked Dr. Nelson for information. Dr. Nelson had read about the beans and explained its health value to Mr. Go. "The bean contains high fiber, protein, folate and minerals. It promotes memory and bone strength." said Dr. Nelson.

Mr. Go got enthusiastic, and though Willie's plant took a little work, he could raise it cheaply. His friend would eat it fresh, and he could dry the rest to sell. He even became more excited when he counted the expected savings from growing it. One acre yielded 2304 pounds. Five acres would yield 11,520 pounds. That equaled a year's supply of food for Willie and some to trade. He decided to grow the plant.

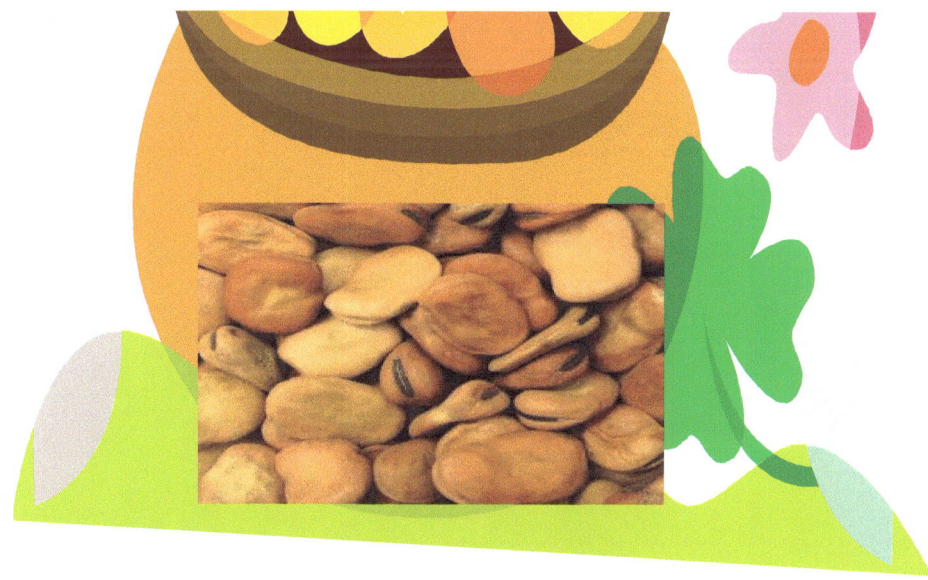

Chris Clark was a second grade neighbor of Mr. Go. He was a healthy, nice but overweight boy who liked candy. His hobby was to grow things. Mr. Go invited Chris to visit his greenhouse after school. Chris liked Mr. Go and enjoyed listening to the stories about his travel adventures. Chris did not do well in school. Kids often joked about his chubby body. Mr. Go knew it troubled his little friend.

During the harvest season, Chris watched Mr. Go loading Willie with the goods to deliver to the stores. As he did every morning, Chris greeted Mr. Go on his way to school.

"Going to the market, Mr. Go?" asked Chris.
"Yes, wish me luck." answered Mr. Go.
"Good luck." said Chris. Each went on his way.

That day, Mr. Go was on foot leading Willie up the hill on their way to the market. Chris noticed that Willie was not his joyous self and thought that Willie must be tired.

Mr. Go saw that, too. He offered Willie his favorite plant, but Willie kept getting weaker. Mr. Go was very displeased with his friend's sudden weakness.

About two miles down the road, Willie was too tired to climb up the hill and cried, "I'm not able to make it."

Then Mr. Go realized that his mule was ill.

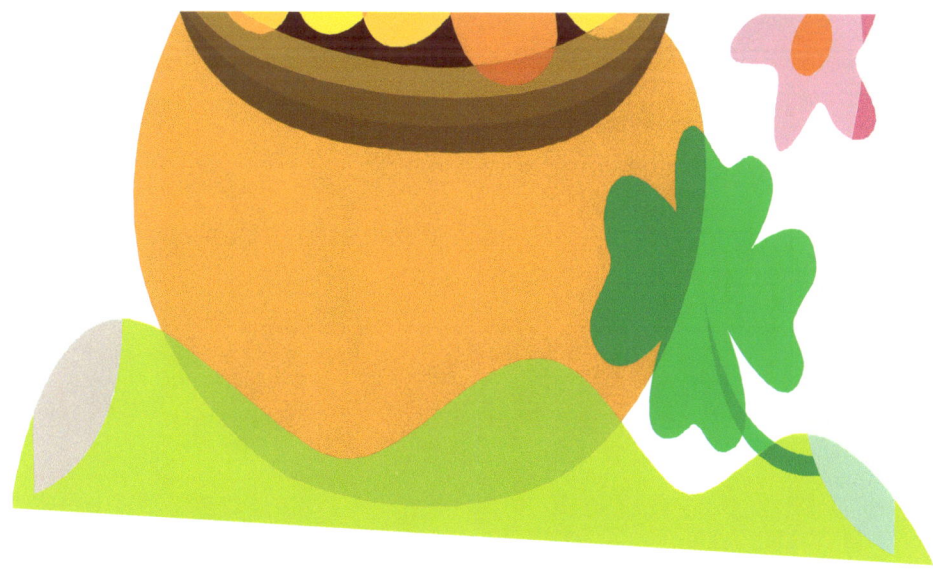

Remember, Mr. Go always thought that his mule was strong. This is why he got puzzled when Willie got sick.

Mr. Go scratched his head for an answer, thinking to himself that Willie might have a cold, and suddenly it occurred to him that the stores were waiting for the goods to be delivered this morning. Mr. Go started to panic.

Down on his knees, he prayed, "Oh God, Willie is my asset. If he could not help me, I will lose my customers. God, cure Willie for me. God, please answer my prayer."

Mr. Go had to quickly figure a way out of his problem and how to keep his business. So he returned Willie to the farm, let him rest and headed to the market to ask store keepers for a day's extension to deliver the goods.

As he was unloading Willie, Mr. Don, a neighbor of Mr. Go, stopped by.
"Need a hand Mr. Go?" asked Mr. Don.
"Yes, would you?" answered Mr. Go.
"You can borrow my donkey, if you tell me the secret," said Mr. Don.
"What secret?" asked Mr. Go.
"The one that made Willie stronger and smarter." said Mr. Don.

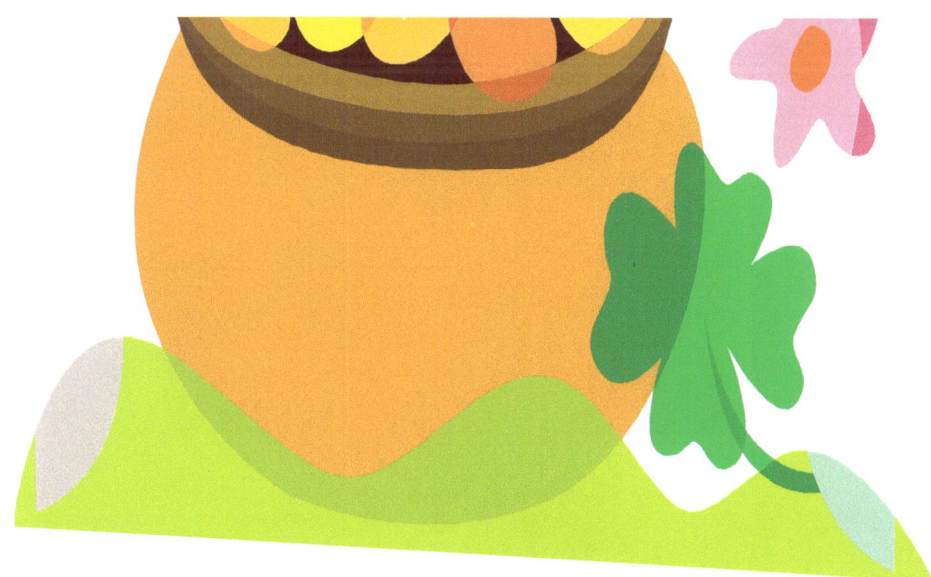

"I wish I knew," answered Mr. Go. Mr. Don was not satisfied with that answer, so he grabbed his donkey and left.

It was an unlucky day for Mr. Go. Things did not go well for him at the market. The shopkeepers did not believe that his mule was ill and would not grant him one more day to make the delivery. Instead, they wanted their money back. But Mr. Go had already used the money, as he did every year, to grow their crops.

The store owners felt cheated and complained to the Mayor.

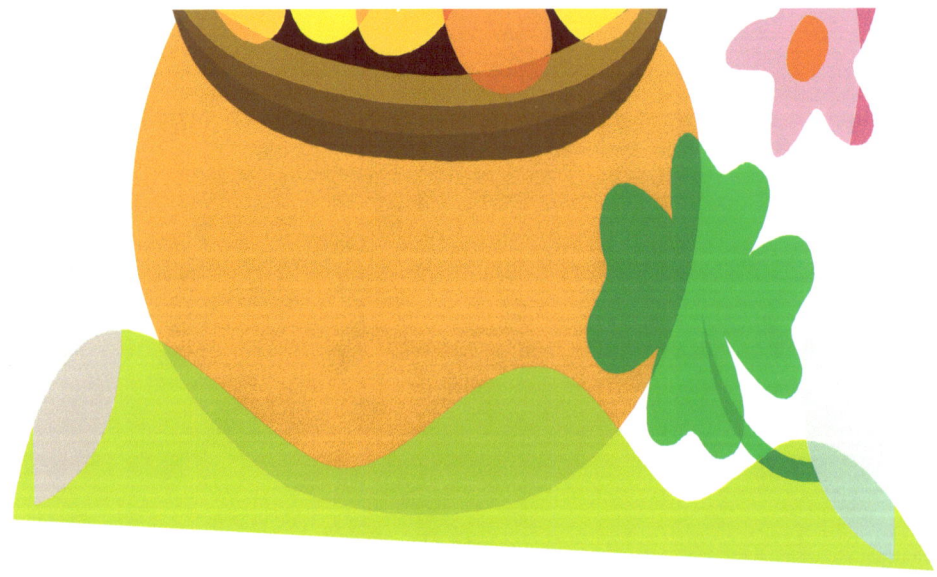

Unfortunately for Mr. Go, Mr. Mayor had back pain that day. He, too, thought that Mr. Go could no longer be trusted and decided to punish him. Mr. Go was deeply saddened for losing his customers' confidence and for getting punished.

Meanwhile, back at the farm, Willie was unloaded and untied. He worked his way to his favorite food. Willie ate and quickly felt so much better.

Again in the mood, Willie was singing his musical to celebrate his returned strength.

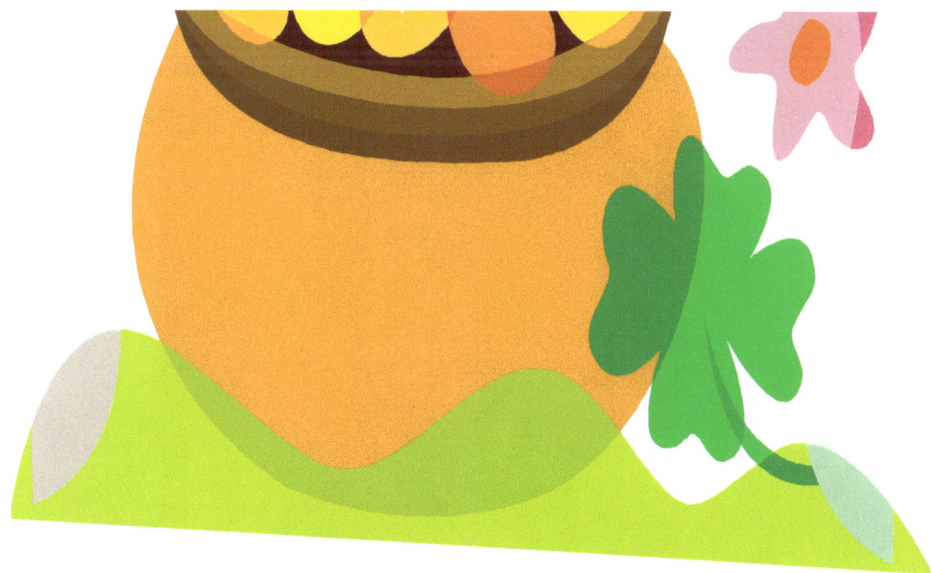

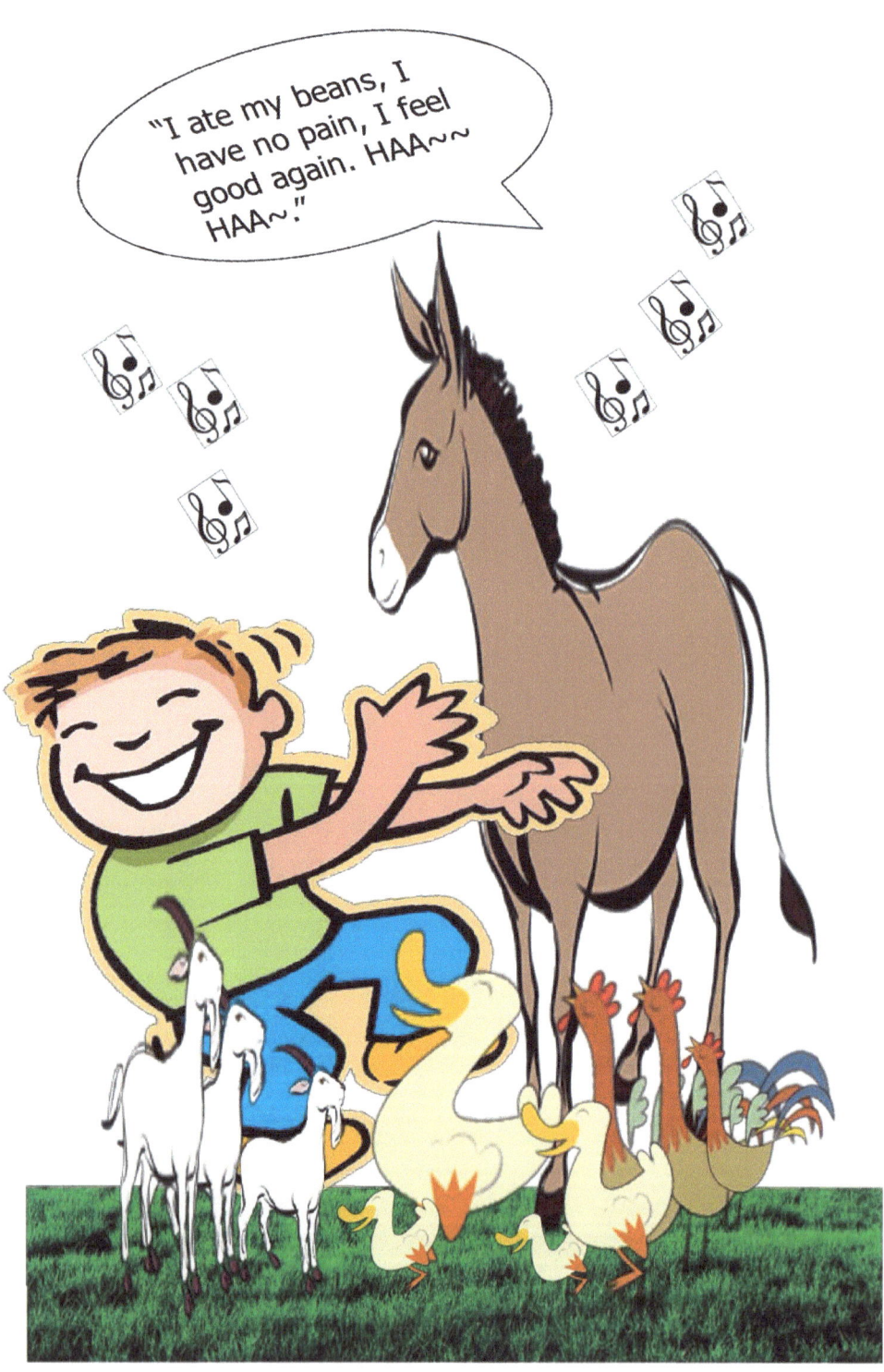

Then all of a sudden, Willie remembered that it was delivery day and that he hadn't yet made it. He stopped singing and screamed, "I let my best friend down. My buddy must be in trouble. In a determined voice shouted Willie "I do not know how, but I'm going to my friend's rescue."

The loyal Willie clicked his hooves and off he rushed up the hill. He travelled the road that he remembered amazingly well on his own.

Willie sang his way into town. "I have no pain! I feel good again! ~~HAA~~HAA~~."

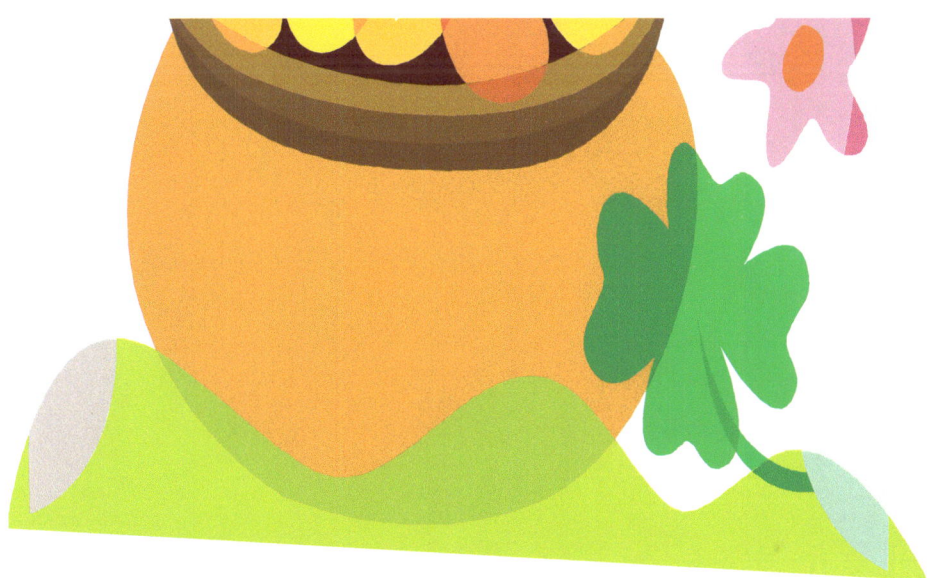

Willie's arrival into town stunned everyone but Mr. Go. He was thrilled to see his friend's quick recovery, although Willie made it without the goods. Shopkeepers who doubted Mr. Go's honesty regretted suspecting him.

Willie's improved health got Mr. Go wondering, "How did Willie regained his strength so quickly, and where did he get the ability to know the way to town by himself?"

"Could it be true that the secret to Willie's healing is in his food, the beans?" Mr. Go thought this must be the magic beans.

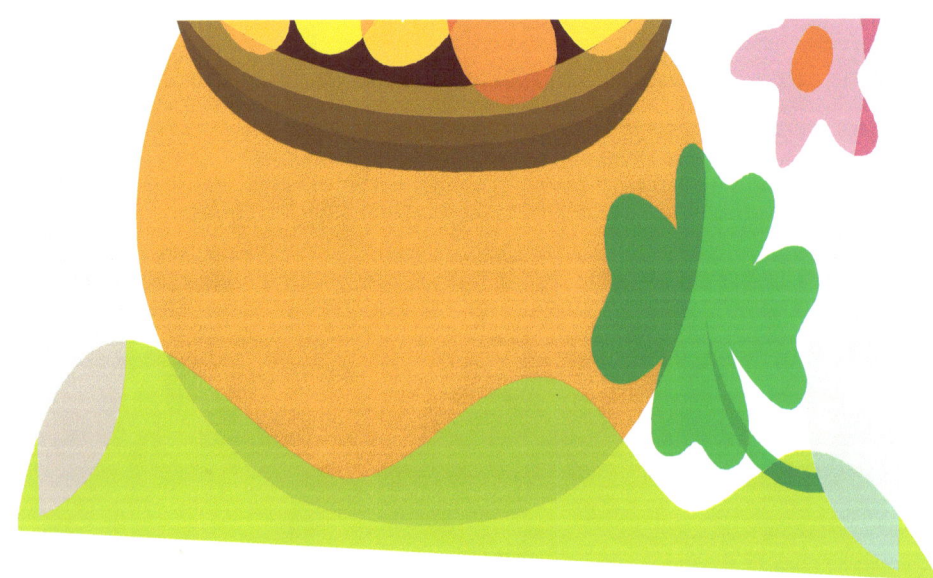

By looking at Willie's condition, Mr. Go became empowered. Once he had discovered the secret of the magic beans, he got a brilliant idea. He said to himself, "If corn was first chicken feed before it became human food, this bean can also become part of man's diet."

Dr. Nelson said that it had health value and it did cure Willie. "Those beans must be the key to make people feel good again, just like Willie."

Mr. Go predicted that the magic beans could be the new health food.

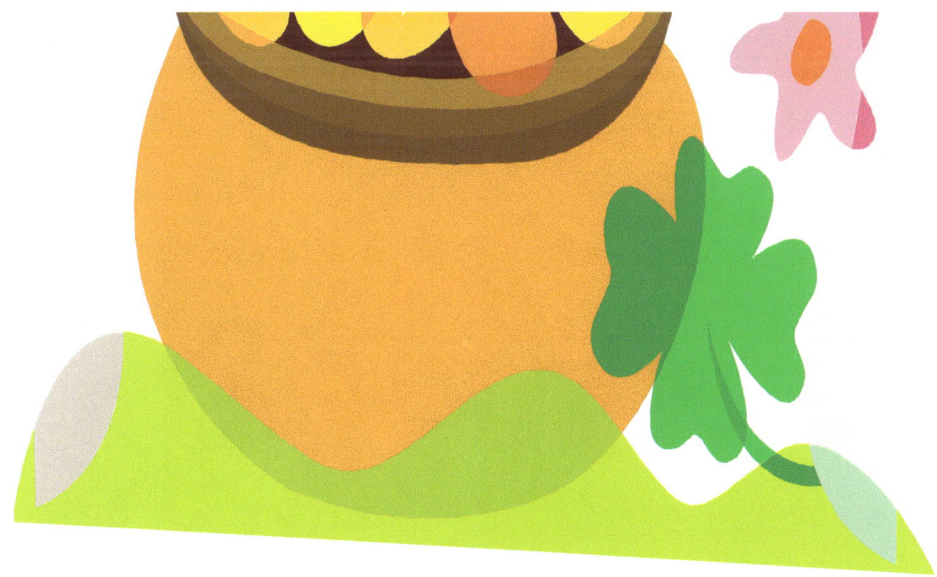

No longer afraid of punishment, Mr. Go made an intelligent move. He proposed to help the Mayor with his health problem.

"Mr. Mayor, I know of a secret solution that I am convinced will help to ease your back pain," said Mr. Go. If my punishment is cancelled and I'm allowed an extension to deliver the goods tomorrow, I will bring you the recipe."

Mr. Mayor accepted his offer.

Shortly after his visit to the market, Mr. Go went back to the farm and called his neighbor, Mr. Don, to announce the good news about the bean discovery and his decision to grow beans for trade. Mr. Don congratulated him and offered to help distribute the crop to the local merchants.

The magic beans became Mr. Go's lucky charm. Farmers bought it he was named the lead bean grower in town and had such success since.

Mr. Go felt it was time to expand the trade and travel abroad to sell the beans in foreign countries.

Mr. Go took a trip across the Atlantic Ocean and headed for the eastern Mediterranean region. The ship arrived a few days later at his first stop, Greece. Mr. Go had a Greek host, a bean merchant named Yanos. He gave Mr. Go a warm welcome and taught him new things about the beans. That it was a popular food among Greeks and that they believed in its health value and antioxidant power. Mr. Yanos reminded Mr. Go about the Hippocratic saying: "Let your food be your medicine, and your medicine be your food."

In Greece, he found many kinds of beans, but with other names like Broad Beans-Fava, Chickpeas-Hummus and Yellow Flat Beans-Luppini. Mr. Go finally found out the name of Willie's plant – Fava beans.

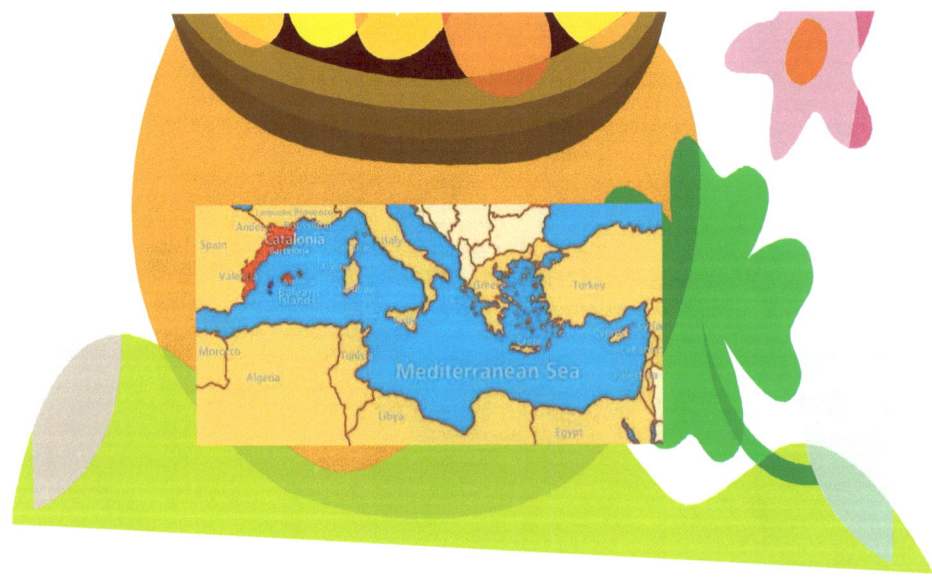

During that season, beans happen to be in short supply on the Greek Islands. So, the merchants bought Mr. Go's crop. It was a fortunate trip for him.

Because he was encouraged with his trip's success, Mr. Go continued fulfilling his life-long dreams. He took a boat to visit the pyramids. South of the Aegean Sea and several hours later, the ship reached the port of Alexandria on the north shore of Egypt. Mr. Go then rode the train to Cairo, his destination. Mr. Solliman, his Egyptian host, was a friendly local bean grower who knew about his guest's interest in health food.

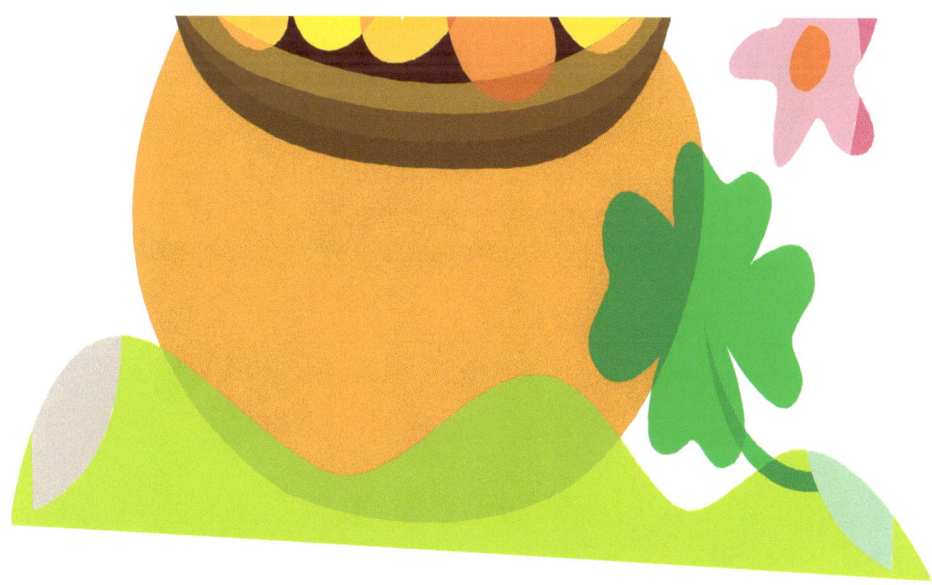

To satisfy Mr. Go's curiosity, Mr. Solliman invited him to food festivals to learn more about beans and taste national dishes.

Mr. Go also attended a folklore re-enactment of treasure-finding where jewelry was replaced by beans.

Mr. Go discovered that beans were the main diet of the people there since 5000 BC as well as the most popular breakfast and baby food.

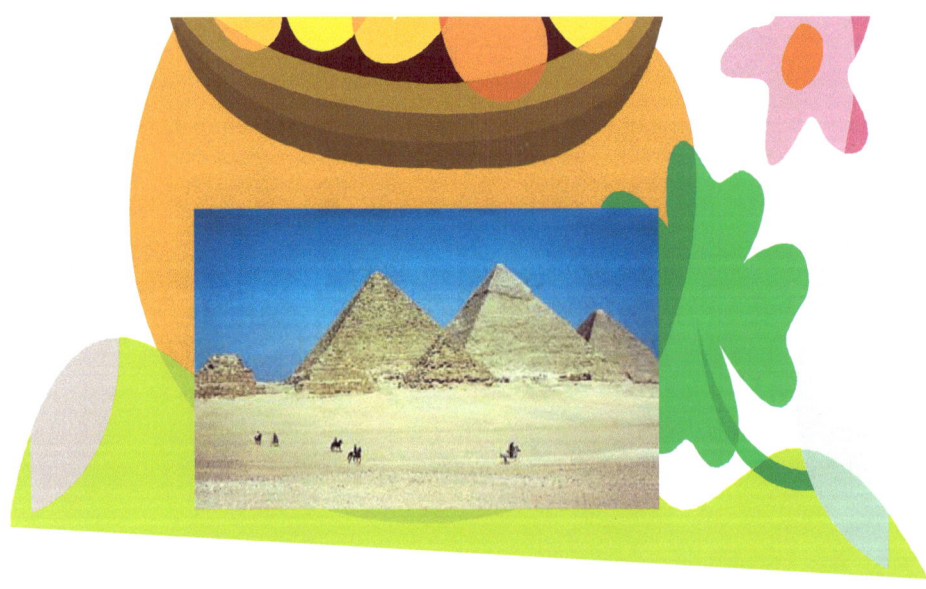

He liked its rich meaty taste and collected beans recipes.

But one question remained unanswered about a song from back home that says "walk like an Egyptian..."

So Mr. Go asked his host, "what about that famous walk? What caused it?"
"The bean diet. It was recorded on ancient scrolls that it balanced nutrition and strengthened bones and memory," said Mr. Solliman.

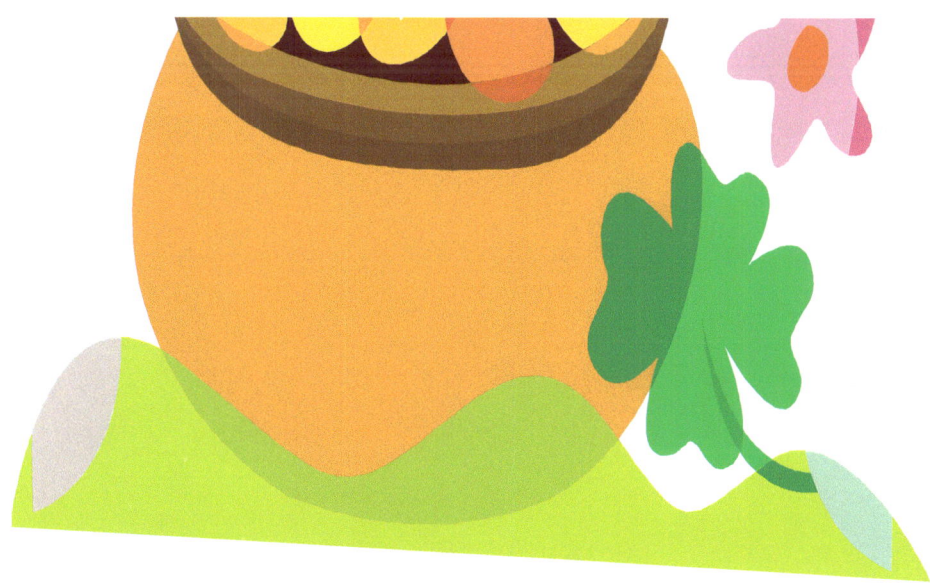

Mr. Go got motivated and thought it would be a real win if he could take this secret recipe back home to help his little friend Chris and to give his son, Dr. Nelson, more ways to assist his patients.

Mr. Go asked his host to help get a translated copy of the scroll. Mr. Solliman did it. Mr. Go returned home victoriously, and his success was celebrated by his community.

Dr. Nelson was especially happy with the scroll. He found more tools to help his patients and to educate them about balanced nutrition. He coordinated with his father to announce the new eating pattern 3-1 to promote normal growth and memory and created a plan to guide parents and teachers.

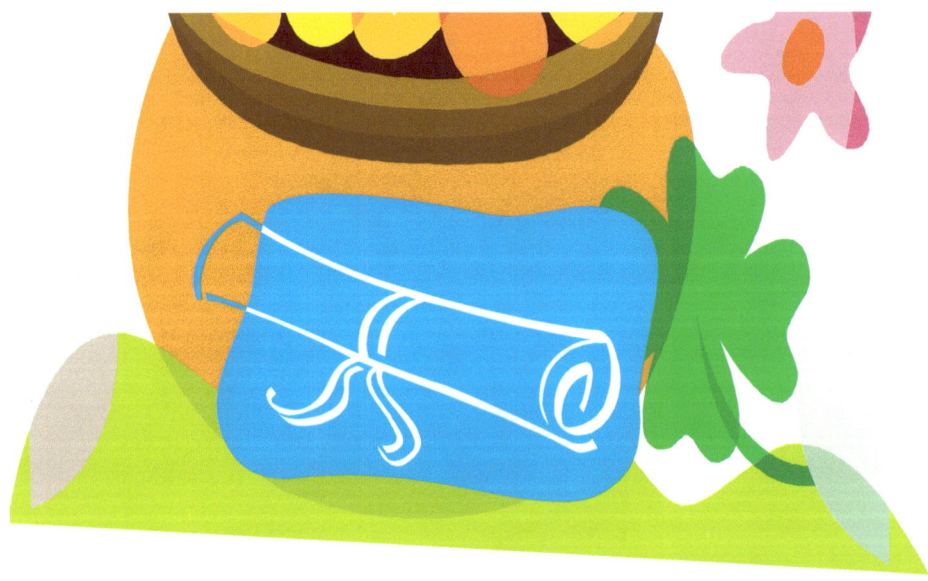

Chris Cark, Mr. Go's buddy, followed the new food diet. He loved the taste so much that he favored this sweet coated bean snack to his old candy. It was even more rewarding for Chris. He slimmed down 20 pounds and felt better about himself because for the first time he got A's and B's in math and science on his report card.

Mr. Go asked Chris "What would you like to be when you grow up?"
"A scientist, answered Chris."

Other children who tried Dr. Nelson's 3-1 model were equally happy. So, Mr. Go named the new diet smart food "Three times smart food meals. One time, other."

The school was very interested in the food that boosts kids' grades and helped heavy children feel better.

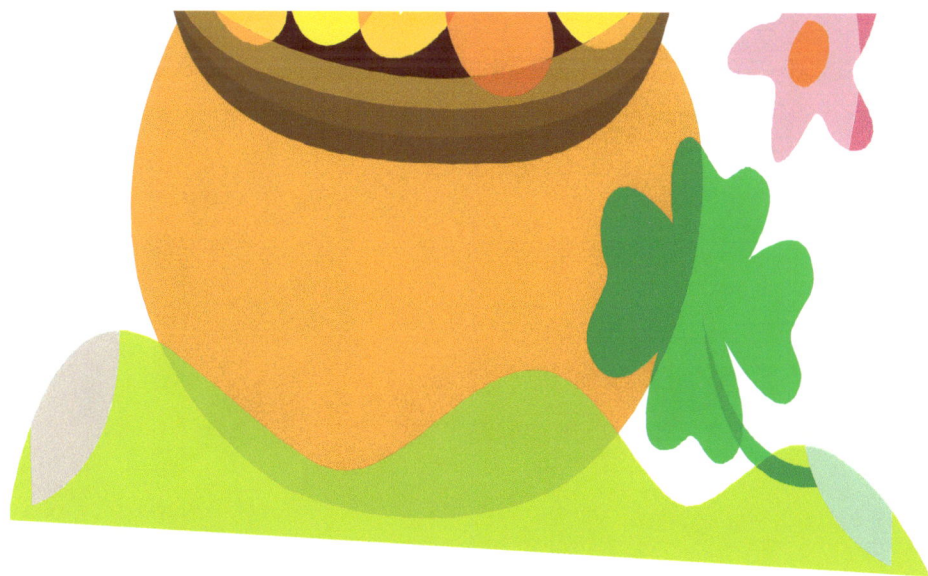

Mr. Go was asked to speak to students about the smart food. Parents were invited, and he called his neighbor, Mr. Don, and the bean merchants to attend. He also asked his son, Dr. Nelson, to help him with the class.

The day of the presentation, Mr. Go gave out a nice gift, knuckle-shaped food calendars. Each contained easy menus of kids' favorites and the smart food pattern so they did not have to make one themselves.

Moms loved the instant bean recipes and teachers found new projects for class.

The Knuckle Calendar

" I enjoy my new food, and I love the beans ' rich meaty taste. "

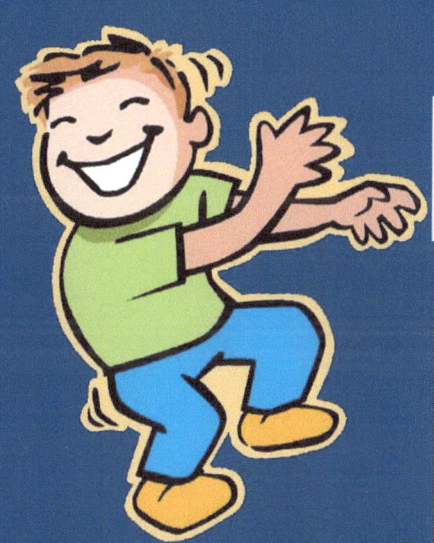

"Three part smart food, one part other."

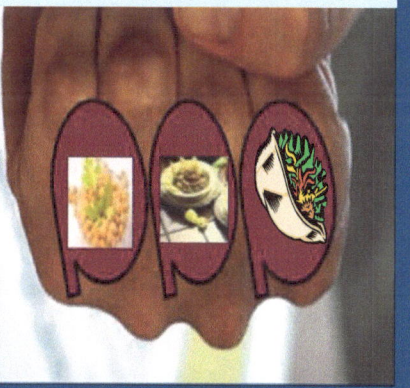

Kids loved the knuckle calendar, learned the smart food 3-1 meals by heart and enjoyed showing off their knowledge. "*Three part smart food, one part other.*"

At the end of his part of the class, Mr. Go asked the kids how they felt about the new food. The kids jumped up, clicked their heels and sang, "I feel good again."

Dr. Nelson took his turn in the class, offering techniques to balance nutrition - boost kids' grades and answering questions.

Mrs. Clark, Chris's mom, was happy with her son's progress and requested information for his siblings.
"How can we improve kid's grades with food?" she asked.

"Use a combination of balanced nutrition, add smart food pattern 3-1 regularly, and provide security for your children," said Dr. Nelson.

"How do I detect imbalance in an infant's diet?" she asked.

"Offer wholesome variety in a suitable form for the child's age and the child will pick what is needed the most." answered Dr. Nelson.

"Is child early aging true?" asked Mrs. Clark.

"Yes," especially among school age kids." said Dr. Nelson.

"What causes it, what are the signs, and what are the risks?" asked Mrs. Clark.

"It is caused by imbalanced nutrition the physical signs include brown skin deposits or molds, white dots on the nails and weakened bones. Other symptoms are lagging memory and mood swings, the risks are that it leads to obesity and unhealthy development." said Dr. Nelson.

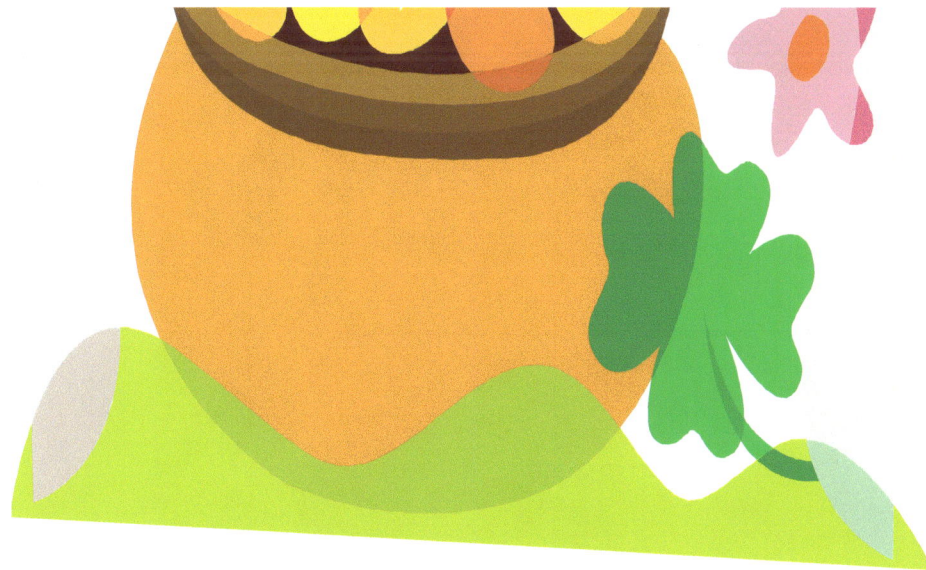

"Can I let my older kids choose their food?" asked Mrs. Clark.

"Yes, and encourage a variety including beans. Report changes to your doctor," advised Dr. Nelson.

After class, the school announced it would hold an Annual Smart Food Contest. The winners Smart King and Queen would be chosen from successful smart and bean diet followers who achieved better grades and improved their body image.

Planning would start right way. Mr. Don and the merchants offered to donate time to support the contest and to participate with Dr. Nelson and the school in the judging panel.

Everyone cheered Mr. Go for inspiring so many good things.

The End

www.ingramcontent.com/pod-product-compliance
Lightning Source LLC
Chambersburg PA
CBHW041533280526
45792CB00004B/1485